AMPHETAMINES AND OTHER STIMULANTS

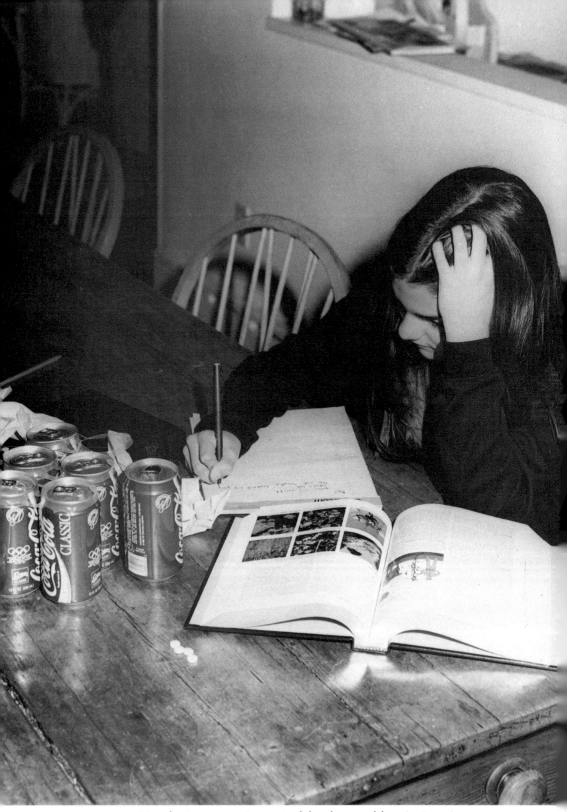

Stimulants are a major part of the drug problem in America.

THE DRUG ABUSE PREVENTION LIBRARY

AMPHETAMINES AND OTHER STIMULANTS

Lawrence Clayton, Ph.D.

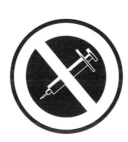

THE ROSEN PUBLISHING GROUP, INC.

NEW YORK

To Annette Colbert, a friend.

The people pictured in this book are only models. They in no way practice or endorse the activities illustrated. Captions serve only to explain the subjects of photographs and do not in any way imply a connection between the real-life models and the staged situations. News agency photos are exceptions.

Published in 1994, 1998 by the Rosen Publishing Group, Inc.
29 East 21st Street, New York, NY 10010

Revised Edition 1998

Library of Congress Cataloging-in-Publication Data

Clayton, L. (Lawrence)
  Amphetamines and other stimulants / by Lawrence Clayton.
    p.   cm. — (The Drug abuse prevention library)
  Includes bibliographical references and index.
  ISBN 0-8239-2584-6
  1. Amphetamines—Juvenile literature. 2. Stimulants—Juvenile
  literature. 3. Drug abuse—United States—Juvenile literature.
  [1. amphetamines. 2. Drug abuse.] I. Title. II. Series.
  HV5822.A5C53 1994
  362.29'9—dc20   94-573
                                                          CIP
                                                          AC

Manufactured in the United States of America

Contents

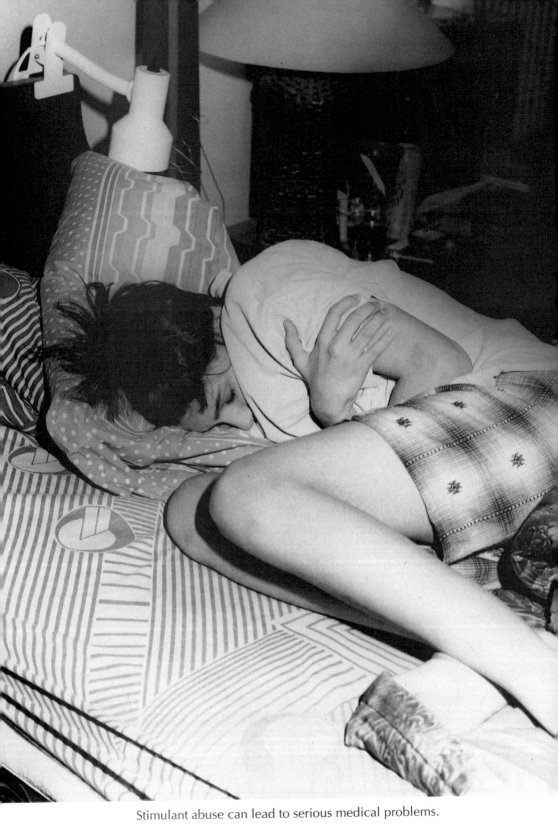

Stimulant abuse can lead to serious medical problems.

Introduction

*J*ana and her friends spent two hours getting ready to go to the new club that had opened downtown. When they got there, it was packed with people dancing. The dance floor was huge, and dozens of colored lights flashed along with the music. It was great, but after an hour or so the crowd and the lights made Jana feel a little tired. She told her friends she was thinking of going home.

"Wait, Jana!" her friend said. "Try this! You'll want to dance all night." Her friend offered her a little white pill. Jana was curious, so she took it.

Suddenly, Jana's heart was pounding. Jana could feel the music throbbing in her

8 | *head. She felt excited and happy at the same time, but her heart was going so fast that she was having trouble breathing.*

Jana is in danger because of the pill she took: an amphetamine. Amphetamines are stimulants, which means that they increase activity in the nervous system.

Amphetamines sometimes are prescribed by doctors to help people with depression, sleep disorders, or severe obesity. But because they can make a person feel alert or happy, amphetamines are regularly abused, especially by teenagers.

Amphetamines are very dangerous if they are abused. They can cause anything from stomach upsets to convulsions to heart problems. When they wear off, amphetamines leave the user exhausted and depressed. In some cases, they even can cause death.

As a teenager, you may have been offered, or may have used, amphetamines. You may just be curious about them. This book will help you find out the facts about amphetamines and other stimulants. You will learn what they are and how they affect you.

This book also will help you learn how you can say no to drugs. If you are already hooked, you can take the first steps toward becoming drug-free. It's never too late to break an addiction and turn your life around.

CHAPTER 1

What Are Stimulants?

*S*timulants (also called "uppers") are drugs that speed up the mind and body. Their effects resemble that of the body's natural hormone adrenalin. But unlike hormones, stimulants can cause serious harm to your body.

Types of Stimulants

Stimulants come in many different forms. The drugs discussed in this book are synthetic, or made in a laboratory. They are generally referred to as amphetamines. But the term "amphetamine" actually refers to several types of stimulants: amphetamines, metham-

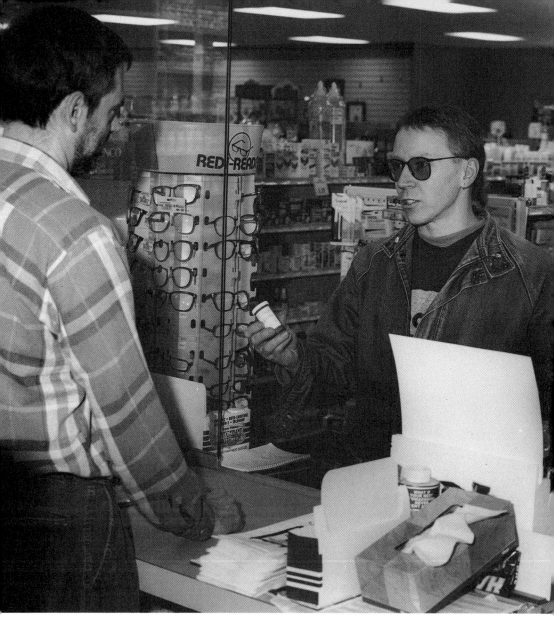

All prescribed medicines should be taken only as directed.

phetamine, and others.

Amphetamines. Amphetamines are drugs sometimes prescribed for weight loss. They also are used to control narcolepsy (a syndrome in which a person will suddenly and uncontrollably fall asleep). They usually are taken in pill form.

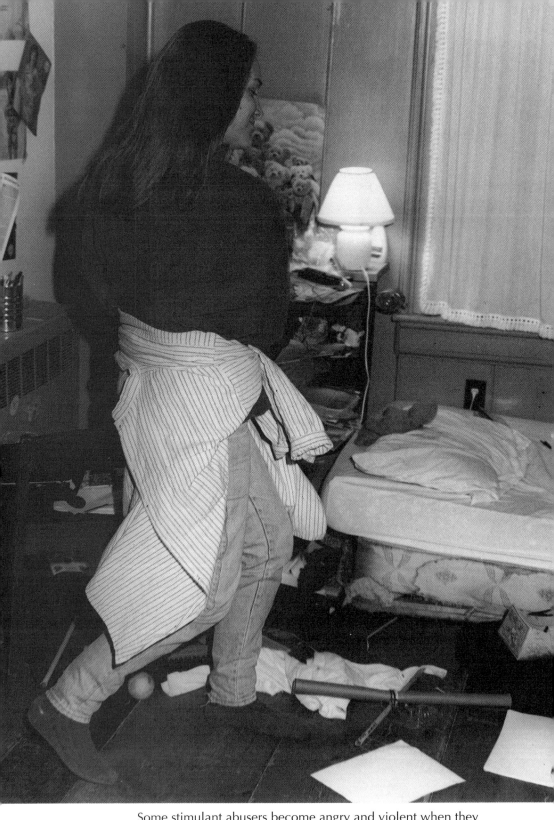

Some stimulant abusers become angry and violent when they are in withdrawal.

Stimulants at a Glance

Amphetamines

Street Names: "speed," "uppers," "pep pills," "hearts," "Black Beauties," "crosses," "bennies," "Mollies," "dexies," "dex," "truck drivers," "ups," "copilots," "footballs," and "go fast."

Trade Names: Biphetamine, Delcobese, Desoxyn, Dexedrine, Obetrol

Methamphetamine

Street Names: "crystal," "go-fast," "meth," "crank," "ice," "glass," "crystal," "zip," "chris," "cristy," "shabu-shabu," "batu."

Trade Names: Benzedrine, Dexedrine, Biphetamine, Metiatric, Obetrol, Desoyxn

Phenmetrazine

Street Names: "phen," "phenz," or "penny."

Trade Name: Preludin

Methylphenidate

Street Names: "rit," "pal," and "lin."

Trade Name: Ritalin

Other Stimulants

Street Names: "ten," "tennies," "two," "Pre," "Cy," "Mel," "Di," "Di-an," "Adi," "T," and "Yellows." Most users simply refer to these drugs as "speed."

Trade Names: Adipex, Cylert, Didrex, Ionamin, Melfiat, Pleigne, Sanorex, Tenuate, Tepanil, Prelu-2

Methamphetamine. This is an extremely potent drug that chemically resembles amphetamines, but is stronger.

Methamphetamine has been used in the past for medicinal purposes. But today it is made mostly in illegal labs by "cooks." Cooking methamphetamine is extremely dangerous: the chemical reactions creates acid fumes that are

14 toxic. Some methamphetamine labs actually have exploded from the fumes coming into contact with a flame.

Methamphetamine can take the form of a fine powder, crystals, or chunks that range in color from off-white to yellow. It can be swallowed, snorted, or injected.

Ice. Ice is a very pure, concentrated form of methamphetamine that looks like tiny chunks of glass ("glass" is another name for it). The drug is "smoked"—vaporized, then inhaled. It is said that as crack is to cocaine, ice is to methamphetamine.

Crystal meth. This drug is among the most abused of all the stimulants because it acts so quickly in the body. The high is almost instantaneous when it is injected into a vein or snorted. The high often is called a "rush" because it is so powerful.

Dealers often mix crystal meth with cocaine or heroin because it is cheaper. Often young people have been given crystal meth believing that they were using cocaine or heroin. This can lead to problems. If a person gets used to taking large doses of crystal meth, and then takes a large dose of straight cocaine or heroin, he or she may overdose.

Phenmetrazine. This drug is pre- scribed by doctors to help people lose weight. It comes only in pill form, and may be swallowed, crushed and snorted, or dissolved and injected into a vein.

Methylphenidate. The trade name for this drug is Ritalin. It is prescribed to calm hyperactive children. When taken in large amounts, this drug acts very much like amphetamines. In some countries methylphenidate can be bought over the counter. In the United States, it is only available by prescription.

The drug is available in pill form. It is usually swallowed, although some users dilute it and inject it into a vein.

Other Stimulants. A few other stimulants have similar effects to amphetamines, but have a different chemical make-up. These "look-alike" drugs can contain different legal substances such as caffeine, ephedrine, and phenylpropanolamine.

Amphetamines and related drugs go by many different names when they are sold on the street. The names can vary by country, by state, and sometimes even by neighborhood. This adds to the problem of amphetamine abuse because a

16 buyer may never really know what he is getting. Each time people buy and use amphetamines, they are taking their lives into their hands.

History of Amphetamines

Amphetamines were first synthesized in 1887. They are drugs that almost didn't get to be drugs—no one could find a use for them until almost 50 years after they were created. Since then, they have been used to treat a variety of problems, from sleep disorders to depression, and in some cases, to help hyperactivity. But in recent decades, they have become widely abused.

A "cure-all." In the 1930s and 1940s, amphetamines were prescribed by doctors. The media labeled amphetamines a "cure-all." Advertisements claimed that amphetamines would solve problems from alcoholism to obesity.

A recreational drug. In the late 1950s, amphetamines were restricted to prescription-only drugs. But people found that the drug was an ingredient in some decongestant inhalers. Students started abusing amphetamines because they helped them stay awake to study. But soon, young people learned that

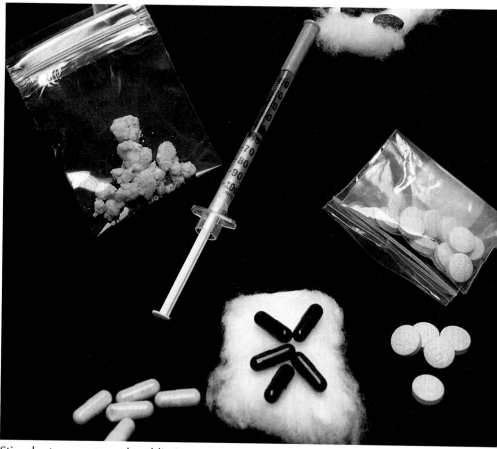

Stimulants are extremely addictive.

large doses produced a euphoric high. Amphetamines then became a popular recreational drug.

Widespread abuse. By the early 1960s, amphetamine abuse was a major problem among young people. Hospitals and doctors began reporting many serious problems: young people were suffering from heart attacks and strokes. This is very unusual for this age group.

17

18   Doctors and pharmacists noticed that young people were forging prescriptions for stimulants. Doctors began to place tighter limits on the amounts of stimulants they prescribed. The police began to crack down on drugstores that sold the drugs illegally.

Speed labs. Soon illegal "speed labs" sprang up on the West Coast. This had many serious consequences. Prescription stimulants were controlled by federal law, but there were no such controls for the illegal labs. Many of them were dirty and did not use trained chemists. Soon hundreds of young people were showing up at hospitals sick or dying from drugs that were made in speed labs.

New drugs. Before long, young people in California found out that mixing heroin with stimulants gave them an unusually intense high. They named this powerful combination a speedball.

Crystal meth became popular in the 1960s as well. When chemists first created this mix, it wasn't a very pure drug, but it gave users the most intense high they had ever experienced.

By the early 1970s, so many people were addicted to stimulants that the United States strictly limited the amounts that doctors could prescribe. As a result, speed labs spread across the country. Soon they were in almost every state.

Looking to the future. One of the biggest dangers of amphetamines and related drugs is that new varieties are created all the time. Throughout the world, centers of the drug culture popularize different "fad" drugs. Some, like crystal meth, have reached epidemic proportions.

You can help end the epidemic by choosing to keep drugs out of your life—for good. Many people choose to stay drug-free after they learn how harmful drugs really are.

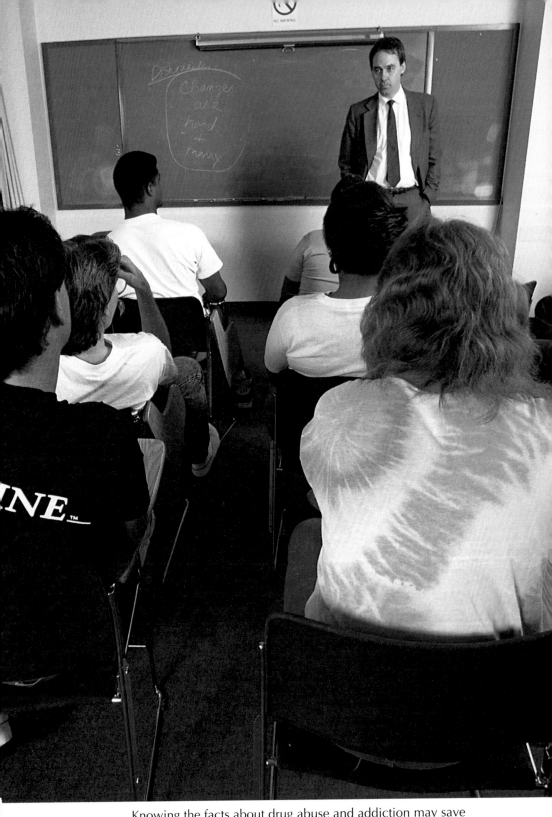

Knowing the facts about drug abuse and addiction may save your life.

CHAPTER 2

The Effects of Stimulants

*M*aalik was a sophomore in high school when he started dating Tonya. She was smart, and had such a strong, positive attitude. In comparison, Maalik felt shy and unsure of himself. He was glad that Tonya had asked him out first, because he wouldn't have been brave enough to do it.

Tonya knew that Maalik was shy, and tried to help. "You know, you have a lot going on inside your head," she told him as they walked home from school. "But you're shy—it's like, you clam up. I wish everyone could see the funny, sweet side of you."

Maalik didn't know how to take that. It seemed like a compliment, but he also

22 | *thought she was calling him a downer.*

Maalik couldn't sleep that night. He felt he had no right to be dragging Tonya down—she deserved a guy who had more to offer. He finally fell asleep at 3AM, after deciding he was going to break up with her.

The next day, Maalik sat down with his friend Tony in the cafeteria. Tony saw how depressed Maalik looked.

"Yo, cheer up, man." Tony punched his arm lightly.

"Cut it out." Maalik didn't look up.

Tony reached into his bag and took out a small plastic packet. He shook some pills out into his hand and handed them to Maalik. "These will give you a jump start," he said. "This round's on me. See you at my party tonight."

Maalik held on to the pills all day. He had refused speed from Tony before, but it felt like he had nothing to lose now. He took them at the end of school, on his way to meet Tonya.

By the time they left school grounds, Maalik was feeling totally revved up. He was talking a mile a minute with Tonya and completely forgot about breaking up with her. When they hit the party, he was laughing and joking with everyone.

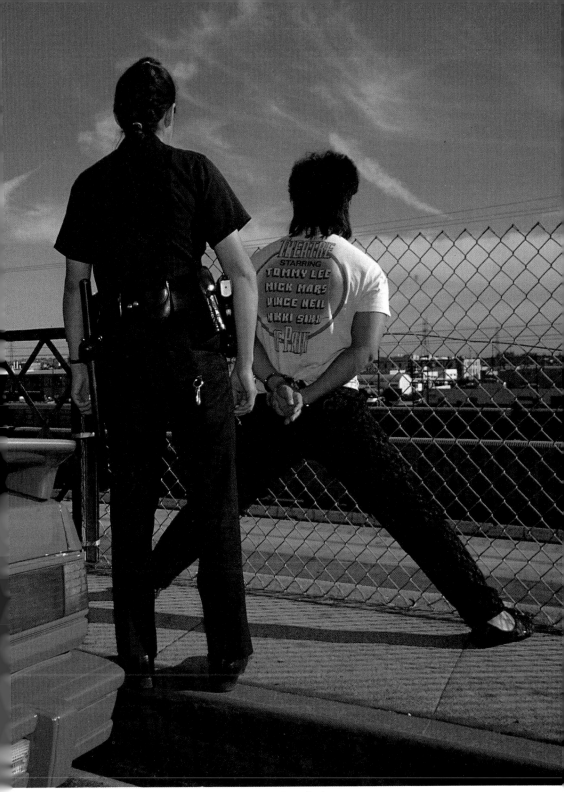

Addicts often turn to crime to support their habit.

24

"Maalik, something's gotten into you tonight," Tonya told him later, pulling him into a corner. "You're really jumpy."

"It's just the 'new me', you know, brand new, starting now!" Maalik gave a high-five to a guy passing by.

"Are you okay? You look kind of pale."

"Look, I'm fine. All right?"

"But Maalik . . ."

"I said stop it!" Maalik slapped her hard.

Short-term Effects

When they are abused, stimulants have many negative effects on your mind and body. They change both how you feel and how you act.

When someone takes stimulants, he or she goes through immediate emotional and physical changes. The first feelings usually are of euphoria, alertness, and energy. But, like Maalik, some users become angry, impatient, and even violent. Other effects include loss of appetite, inability to sleep, and mood swings.

Physical changes occur as well. Users have headaches, chest pain, enlarged pupils, or sudden movements. They also may talk very fast, have a dry mouth, and clench or grind their teeth.

Stimulants also can kill you instantly. Just one dose can cause heart failure, very high fever, or a burst blood vessel in the brain.

It is especially dangerous to use stimulants when exercising. Physical exertion causes one's blood pressure and heart rate to increase. The stimulants have already increased the blood pressure and heart rate, so a stroke or heart attack can result from this overexertion.

Long-term Effects

The long-term effects of using stimulants also are devastating. They include weight loss, a rash that looks like chicken pox, boils, gum disease, distorted vision, lung problems, uncontrollable shaking, and brain damage.

There are many other dangers. Users may suffer from fever, convulsions, high blood pressure, depression, severe fatigue, intense anger, nausea, vomiting, stomachaches, paranoia, blackouts, suicidal tendencies, coma, and even death.

Kellie had been given a prescription for weight-loss pills a year ago. She had been eighty pounds overweight, and was thrilled

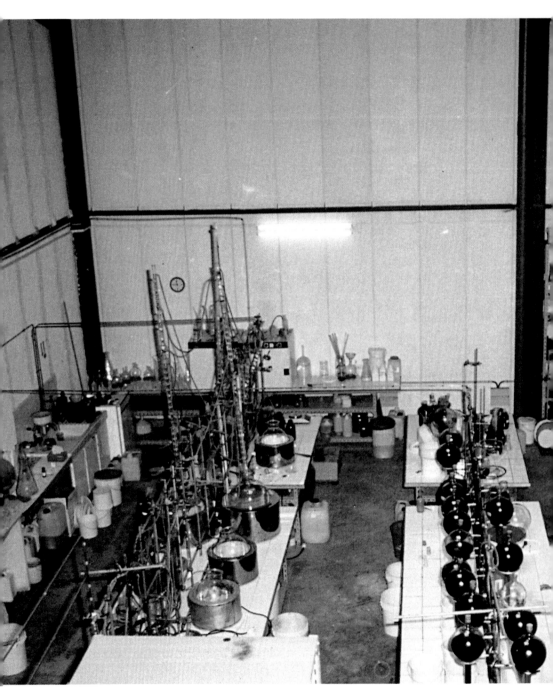

Drugs produced in an illegal lab can be deadly poison.

when the pounds seem to melt away.

Kellie continued to take the drug over the course of several months. But after awhile the pounds stopped coming off. Kellie's doctor told her that her body had reached a set point. "You shouldn't try to be stick thin," she told Kellie. "You're at a point now where you can maintain a healthy weight through diet and exercise."

Kellie was devastated. She felt that she had to keep losing weight no matter what. When Kellie's doctor took her off the pills, Kellie tried some over-the-counter diet drugs. But soon she wanted something stronger.

Kellie started buying methamphetamine from an acquaintance at school. She continued to lose weight. But she also had rashes on her skin, and starting flying into rages for no reason. Her parents called an ambulance one night when Kellie was hallucinating scorpions crawling up the walls.

Kellie is still in the hospital. The doctors say that her chronic use of methamphetamine may have given her permanent brain damage.

Stimulant Addiction

Stimulants create a cycle of feelings and behavior in users. The high can be very strong, and users believe that they can do anything.

A stimulant high is followed by a crash. The drug wears off, and the user often will become depressed. A person will then use stimulants again in order to bring on another high.

This cycle of getting high and crashing puts a person on the road to addiction. Addiction is loss of control over use of a drug. Once you start using stimulants, you crave them and use them until you can't function without them.

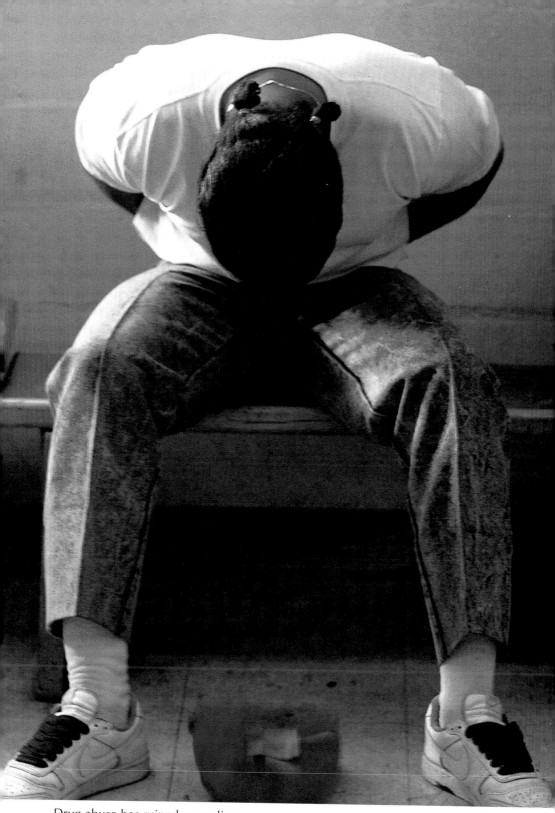

Drug abuse has ruined many lives.

30　　Addiction can be both physical and psychological. A user can psychologically depend on the high brought on by stimulants. She can become physically addicted because she will develop a tolerance to the drug, needing larger and larger doses in order to get the same high.

People sometimes use stimulants over and over without even stopping, even to sleep. Users call this "going on a run" or "tweaking." When they finally do stop using, they come down off the high even harder. Then they can become very angry, hostile, and depressed.

Withdrawal

If people who are addicted to stimulants can't get drugs, they go into withdrawal. The signs of withdrawal include depression, paranoia, long periods of sleep, anger, constant hunger, lack of energy, and violence. Withdrawal is so difficult, addicts will do almost anything to get more drugs: they may rob people, write bad checks, or shoplift. Fifty percent of violent crimes are committed when the offender is under the influence of drugs.

When you choose to stop using stimulants, it's important that you do it safely. You can handle the symptoms of withdrawal if you have support and the facts. Talk to your parents, a friend's parents, a drug counselor, teacher, or guidance counselor. If you don't feel comfortable talking to any of them, contact one of the organizations listed in the back of this book. There are people out there who want to help you.

Addiction Is a Process

What if you're not sure whether you really are addicted to stimulants? You may have tried speed at a party. You may have used drugs off and on, whenever you run into someone who is selling them. You think you have everything under control. But do you?

The scary thing about addiction is that that it happens without realizing it. Like other addictions, stimulant addiction occurs in stages.

Stage I: Experimenting. *When Amie started eighth grade, she felt lonely and tried hard to make new friends. She was thrilled when LaDawn, one of the girls in her science class, asked her to come over after school. Amie was especially glad because her own home was a war zone:*

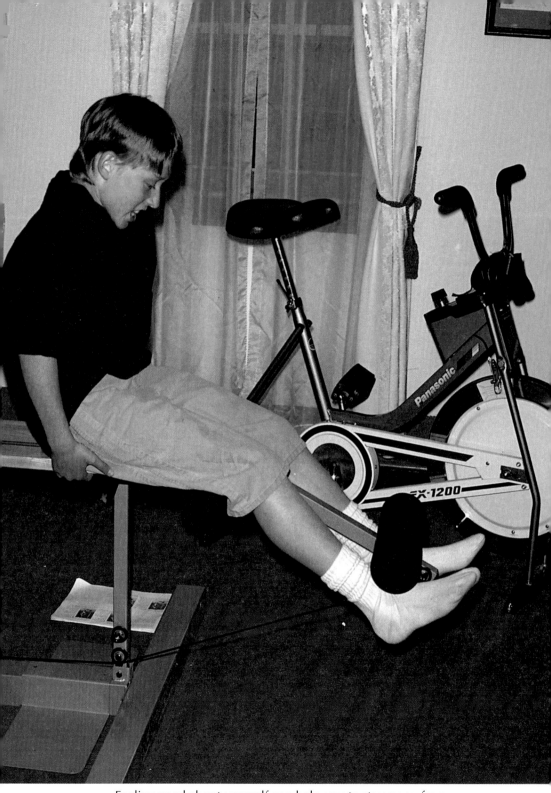

Feeling good about yourself can help you to stay away from drugs.

her mom and dad were fighting all the time.

Amie and LaDawn became close friends. They also started experimenting with drugs together. First they tried sniffing glue. They also stole some marijuana from LaDawn's older sister. Amie's younger brother had a prescription to treat hyperactivity. Amie and LaDawn found that when they took the pills, they got a high.

Amie and LaDawn did not take their drug use very seriously. They were just looking for something to do, and used whatever was around. But things soon started to get out of hand.

Stage 2: Regular Use. *Amie and LaDawn started making new friends. Jake's family was pretty well off— his parents frequently were out of town on business trips, and let him stay home alone. Jake invited Amie and LaDawn over a lot, along with some other neighborhood kids. Amie and LaDawn told them that they were getting high from this prescription drug. Jake knew someone who sold it illegally at school. Soon that was the only drug they used.*

Amie still didn't think much of her drug use. She was grateful to have a place to

34 | *hang out in the afternoons. The drug made her feel alert and happy. In comparison, when she was at home, all she wanted to do was cry. She began to crave the next high.*

Stage 3: Harmful Involvement. *Amie started staying high for long stretches of time. Her parents didn't seem to notice. The drug dealers at school turned her on to a few different drugs. She found some that were much more powerful than what she had been using.*

Amie's friends knew that her home life was a nightmare. But when Amie didn't come to school, they got worried. Sometimes Amie would drop by Jake's house, ringing the doorbell in the middle of the night. She would talk constantly for an hour, start to come down, sleep for about twelve hours, and disappear while Jake was at school.

LaDawn tried talking to Amie. But Amie didn't want to hear any of it, and screamed that LaDawn was spying on her. LaDawn didn't know where her old friend had gone. Privately, she decided never to touch drugs again—she didn't want to become like Amie.

Stage 4: Chemical Dependence. *Amie's health declined rapidly. She lost a*

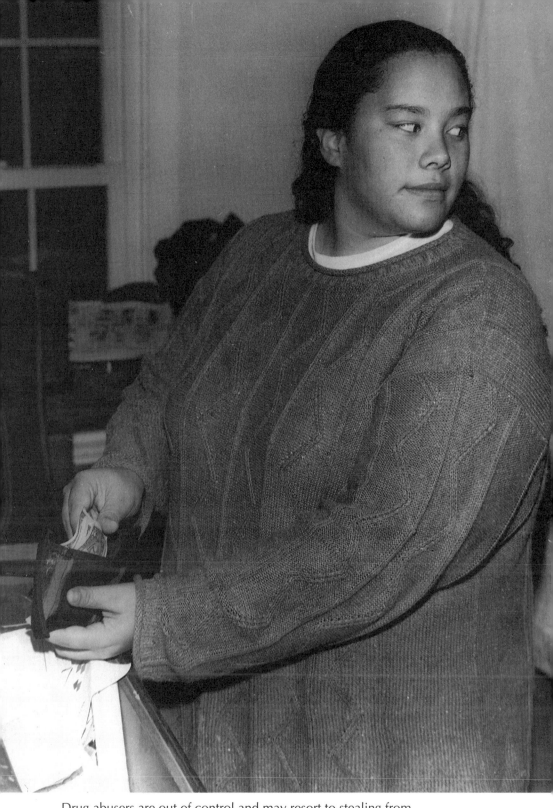

Drug abusers are out of control and may resort to stealing from their own family.

36

lot of weight. Sometimes she hallucinated imaginary spots on her skin and began picking at them. She stayed awake for days at a time.

Amie knew she was out of control, but she couldn't stop.

The time it takes to go through these stages is different for each person. It took Amie only a few months to become addicted to stimulants.

Are you wondering whether you have a drug problem? Ask yourself a few questions:

- Do you worry about your drug use?
- Do you tell lies to cover up your drug use?
- Do you feel like you can't get through the day without drugs?
- Do you have bouts of exhaustion or insomnia because of your drug use?
- Has your appetite been affected because of your drug use?
- Are you having other physical problems as a result of your drug use?

If you answer "yes" to any of these questions, you are at risk for stimulant addiction. Please keep reading and find out how you can reach out for help.

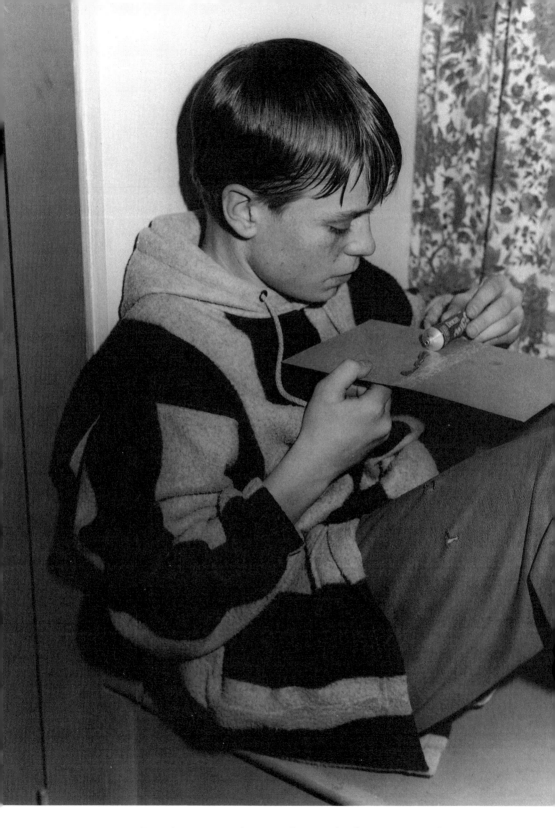

Experimenting with many drugs is the first step toward addiction.

CHAPTER 4

Why People Abuse Stimulants

You may turn to drugs to ease conflict and unhappiness. You also may be reacting to stressful situations in your life.

Everyone has a different reason for turning to drugs. But most people have one thing in common: the drug use is only part of the problem.

Looking at your emotions and the world around you is an important part of dealing with a drug problem. Maybe you will see yourself in this chapter.

Loneliness

Diana's family moved to a new city three months ago. It was hard for all of

39

40 *them, but Diana was having a lot of trouble adjusting. Back home, she'd known everyone, and she'd been popular with everyone. She knew all the best places to hang out, and always had friends who wanted to hang out with her.*

One night, Diana decided to go out on her own and try to make some new friends. But everyone was with other people that they knew well. No one even approached her to talk. Diana quickly walked to the bathroom so no one would see the tears in her eyes.

A girl in the bathroom saw Diana crying and put a comforting hand on her shoulder. "Hey, don't be so sad. Here, take this, it'll make you feel a lot better." She handed Diana a small, oval pill.

"Who knows what this could do to me," Diana thought, "but who cares? I'm all alone anyway."

Family Problems

Lee couldn't stand it anymore. His mom had taken off again. Sometimes she would be gone for days, and since Lee's dad had died two years ago, Lee would have to take care of his two younger sisters.

Lee didn't know how he could deal with all of this responsibility. Plus, he would have to deal with his mom when she got home. Lee knew that when his mom disappeared, it usually meant she was on a drinking binge.

Lee was tired all the time from all the pressure and responsibility he felt. He started falling asleep in school. But one of his friends turned him onto a drug that would keep him awake: crystal meth. Lee started using it every day. Then he could do all his chores and not feel tired.

By the time Lee's mom came home drunk, Lee had been up for three days straight. Lee flew into a rage and knocked his mother to the ground.

Lee had started taking drugs because he felt pressure to hold the family together. But because of Lee's drug use, his problems were getting worse.

There are many reasons why addiction can go hand in hand with family problems. Teens may turn to drugs to escape unhappiness at home. Also, in some families, drugs may be abused by a parent. Parents may even supply their teenagers with drugs, or leave the drugs where the teens can find them.

Drug abuse may be a family's way of coping with problems. Some families

42 never talk about or deal with problems. Instead, they turn to drugs in order to forget. But it really makes things worse.

Depression

You probably have felt "down in the dumps" or "blue" at different times in your life. It's normal to feel this way once in a while. You may have broken up with a boyfriend or girlfriend, or lost a big game. Usually the hurt passes, and life goes on.

But what if the feeling just doesn't go away? You may not want to eat, or even get out of bed. You may have trouble concentrating, and feel hopeless most of the time. You may even have thoughts of hurting yourself or others. When your feelings are this strong, you may be suffering from depression.

Depression is a common psychological disorder that can be treated. The best way to get help is to approach a counselor at school, or tell your parents. Sometimes it helps to talk to a therapist about your feelings. If you find you need additional help, there are several medications that a doctor or psychiatrist can prescribe for you.

You *never* should use amphetamines

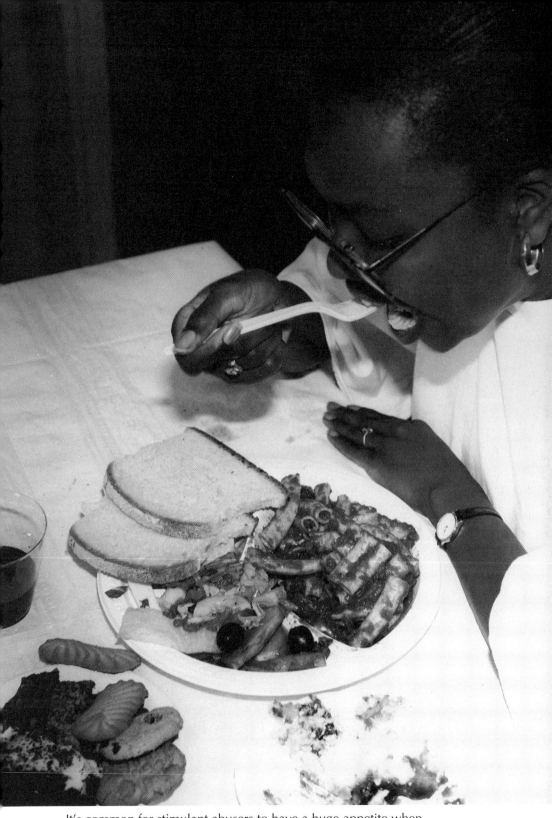

It's common for stimulant abusers to have a huge appetite when they stop taking drugs.

44 | and other stimulants in order to treat depression yourself. They can only make your symptoms worse, because every high is followed by a crash. If you and your doctor decide to treat your depression with medication, many different kinds of medication can help. Work together with your doctor to find which one works best.

One of the best things you can do is talk about your feelings, and what's going on in your life, with someone who will listen. Find someone close to you that you can trust.

CHAPTER 5

Breaking Addiction

*D*rug abuse is a very difficult problem to tackle. For many abusers, the hardest part is admitting that they need help. Most drug abusers think that the drugs help them to be a better person—they think they are more capable, more social, and more successful when they are high, so they cannot imagine being sober.

Drug abusers think that without their drug, they will be unable to continue their daily lives. But that isn't true at all.

Getting Help

Some people think that they can kick their drug habit on their own. They may be embarrassed to get outside help, or

46 they may feel as though its no one's business but their own.

But drug addiction has to be treated physically *and* mentally. The body needs to detoxify, or get rid of the drug. Sometimes a stay in a hospital or clinic is needed in order to detoxify. This is normal. And it helps to have people around you who are struggling with the same kinds of problems you are.

Getting off drugs can be painful, both physically and mentally. Having others around to help you will increase your chances of successfully kicking the habit. There are a number of drug treatment options available for those who are ready to get help.

Personal Counseling

A personal counselor is someone you can talk to about your problems. Counselors can help you start to think about why you're using drugs, and help you identify real solutions to your problems. You can talk honestly with a counselor without having to worry about hurting his or her feelings, or about what he or she will think of you.

Counselors can't discuss what you tell them with other people, so it's safe to

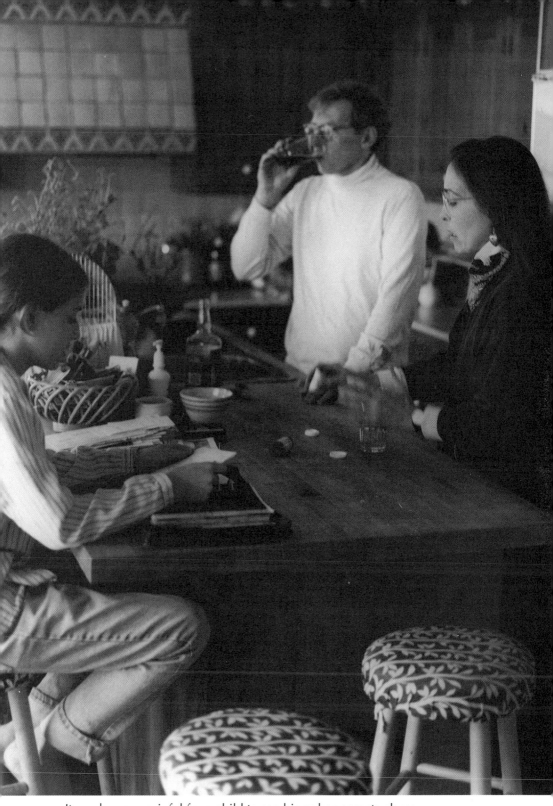

It can be very painful for a child to see his or her parents abuse
drugs.

48 | talk about anything that's on your mind.

Self-Help Groups

Self-help groups usually have three or four goals that members want to achieve, such as learning how to manage emotions and behavior in ways that are healthy.

The groups focus on giving members the tools they need to deal with their problems and urges. Group sessions help members feel confident that they don't need a drug to get through hard times— they will have the personal power and support to face problems.

Self-help groups can be found in the Yellow Pages, in the newspaper, or on the World Wide Web.

Twelve-Step Programs

Twelve-step programs, such as Alcoholics Anonymous, have been very successful at helping people stay drug-free.

Twelve-step groups help people develop the tools they need to stay sober. Members work through twelve specific steps toward recovery, beginning by admitting that they have a problem. Meetings are free and open to anyone struggling with addiction.

Twelve-step programs also can be

found in the newspaper, in the phone book, or on the World Wide Web.

How to Choose What's Best for You

People will need different kinds of support in order to kick their habit.

Some people feel more supported in self-help groups or twelve-step programs, because they are meeting others who are in the same situation they are in. Others need individual attention because they don't feel comfortable discussing their personal life with a group. Some teens may feel that an adult cannot understand what they're going through, and may instead meet with a peer counselor.

Some people believe that just talking to friends will help them kick their drug habit. But a friend may not have the resources or experience to provide you with the best advice. A professional can help you deal with the problems that are making you feel that drugs are a solution.

Expectations

Getting off drugs is more than just a single action—it's a process. It involves

50 | actually stopping the physical use of the drug. But it also involves getting to the root of why your drug problem began in the first place. In the last chapter, we discussed some of the reasons people abuse drugs. It's often because of other issues in their lives.

Part of drug treatment is figuring out what those issues are, and learning to deal with them constructively. It takes time. It's important to be realistic about just how much time it will take to figure out those problems. Setting unreasonable expectations for yourself can make you depressed when you find that you're unable to meet them. And that can bring you back to the kind of situation that led to your drug use in the first place. Give yourself time to really recover from your addiction, so you can move forward with confidence.

It can be tough to go from rehabilitation back into a social life. Others seem to be using drugs without any problems. But a combination of determination and support from family, friends, and other sources can help you stick to your recovery.

The recovery process is a long one.
But it helps to remember that recovery
is helping you regain control of your life.

51

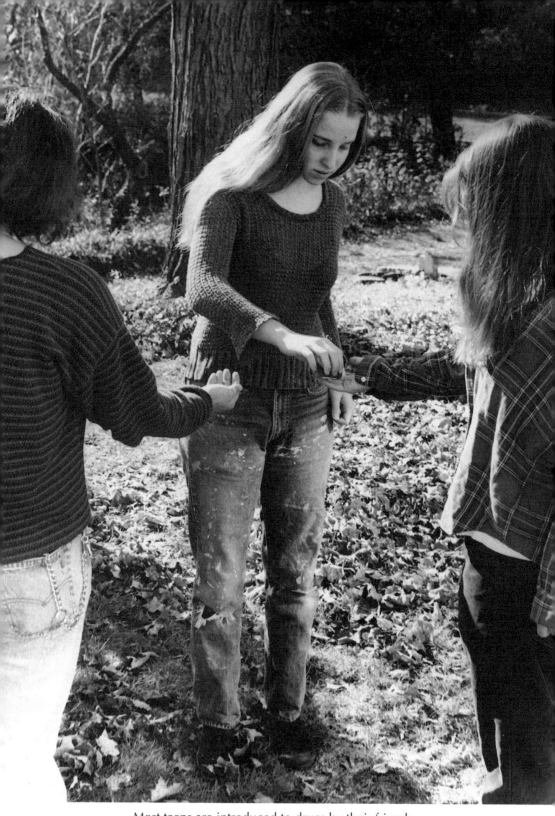

Most teens are introduced to drugs by their friends.

CHAPTER 7

Beating Peer Pressure

*P*eer pressure is a major reason young people get hooked on drugs. Your peers are other people your age. For our purposes, peer pressure means pressure to use drugs. Your friends may try to convince you that using stimulants will make you happy in a way that you wouldn't be otherwise.

Sources of Peer Pressure

As a teen, you are facing peer pressure all around you. It comes from many different sources.

Wanting to be cool. The words change, but the idea is that you want the other kids to respect you. But where does respect come from? It starts with self-respect. Would you respect someone

53

54 who didn't respect him- or herself?

Do you respect people who use drugs? Would others respect you if you used drugs? How would you feel about yourself if you became addicted?

Fear of criticism. Let's face it: no one likes to be criticized. Being made fun of can be painful.

But what do teens think of those who use drugs? Do they make friends of the speed freaks, or the "stoners"? Or do they criticize them?

Pressure from dealers. Some people get addicted to drugs because dealers (sometimes called "pushers") pressure them. The dealers are very good at that. They can make you feel stupid or weak if you don't try drugs.

Dealers have many ways to get teens hooked on drugs. It is their job. They may threaten to hurt you or someone you care about. They may give you free samples. They will do whatever they can to get you hooked. Once you're addicted, they know you'll buy again and again.

Beating Peer Pressure

We have talked about why peer pressure can be hard for you. Now let's look

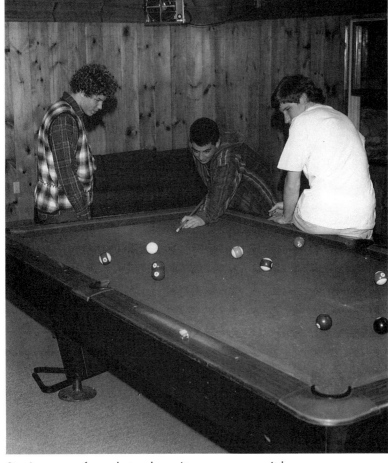
Staying away from drugs doesn't mean you can't have a good time.

at ways you can beat peer pressure.

Know yourself. It is important to have a sense of who you are. Psychologists call this "a sense of identity." It means knowing what you want out of life. Do you want to be an airline pilot, an army officer, or a senator?

Drugs could ruin your chance to be any of those things. If you know who you are and what you want, it will be hard for anyone to push you into taking drugs.

Have a long-range view. That means

56 | seeing the big picture. Have you ever seen a movie about someone's life? If you could see a movie of how things were going to turn out for you, would it affect the way you live today? Of course it would! If you knew you were going to have an unsuccessful career because you used drugs when you were young, would you use them anyway? If you knew that you would become permanently paralyzed after a bad dose of drugs, would you continue to use them? If you knew that drugs would kill parts of your brain every time you used them, would you go on?

If you have a long-range view, you can see that using drugs hurts your chances of success in life. Counselors often refer to addicts as "chronic underachievers." This means that they never get as far as they could have.

Be assertive. This means telling people what you want and what you do not want. It means saying no and meaning it. It means refusing to use drugs or ending your use. Assertiveness can be difficult at first, but it gets easier with practice.

When you first use assertiveness, drug dealers will try to make you give in. If you continue to say no, they will leave you alone.

Ask an adult's advice. Parents and
other adults can help you find ways to
deal with peer pressure. Pastors, rabbis,
teachers, and grandparents have had
years of experience in dealing with things
like peer pressure. (Yes, even they had
problems with peer pressure.) You may
be surprised how well their advice
works.

Amphetamines and other stimulants
are very dangerous substances. When
you're feeling depressed or overwhelmed,
the kind of effects which they promise
can seem appealing. But the long-term
effects can be devastating.

You have alternatives—and you have
the right to say no to drugs.

Glossary
Explaining New Words

abuse Use of a drug in a manner other than how it is prescribed.

addiction State or condition of being unable to stop using a drug.

coma A state of unconsciousness as a result of disease or poison.

convulsion Involuntary and violent spasm of the muscles.

crash The depression that hits stimulant abusers when coming down from a high.

crystal-meth Street name for combination of methedrine and amphetamine; also called methamphetamine.

detox The process of removing drugs from the body.

dose Amount of a drug used at one time.

euphoria An exaggerated feeling of well-being that has no basis in reality. **59**

hallucination Something seen or felt that does not exist outside the mind; sometimes called a "wandering of the mind."

run Period of several days of drug use without sleep.

seizure A spasm of the body.

speed Slang for drugs that excite the mind and body.

speedball A combination of speed and heroin.

tweaking Another term for "going on a run;" using stimulants over and over without stopping.

uppers Drugs that excite the mind and body; also called *speed*.

withdrawal The physical effects of being without drugs.

Where to Go for Help

American Council for Drug Education
204 Monroe Street
Rockville, MD 20852
(301) 294-0600

American Self-Help Clearinghouse
http://www.cmhc.com/selfhelp

Just Say No International
2000 Franklin Street
Oakland, CA 94612
(800) 258-2766

National Council on Alcoholism and
    Drug Dependence
12 West 21st Street
New York, NY 10010
(800) 622-2255
web site: http://www.ncadd.org/
e-mail: national@NCADD.org

National Federation of Drug-Free Youth
8730 Georgia Avenue
Silver Springs, MD 20910

National Institute on Drug Abuse (NIDA)
5600 Fishers lane
Rockville, MD 20857
(800) 662-HELP
web site: http://www.nida.nih.gov

Youth Crisis Hot Line
(800) 448-4663

For Further Reading

Ball, Jacqueline A. *Everything You Need to Know About Drug Abuse*. New York: Rosen Publishing Group, Inc., 1994, rev. ed.

McCormick, Michelle. *Designer-Drug Abuse*. New York: Franklin Watts, 1989.

Seymour, Richard, et. al. The New Drugs: Look-Alikes, Drugs of Deception, and Designer Drugs. Center City, MN: Hazelden Foundation, 1989.

Strazzabosco-Hayn, Gina. *Drugs and Sleeping Disorders*. New York: Rosen Publishing Group, 1996.

Challenging Reading

Myers, Arthur. *Drugs and Emotions*. New York: Rosen Publishing Group, 1996.

Index

About the Author

Dr. Lawrence Clayton earned his doctorate from Texas Woman's University. He is an ordained minister and has served as such since 1972. Dr. Clayton is a clinical marriage and family therapist and certified drug and alcohol counselor. He is also president of the Oklahoma Professional Drug and Alcohol Counselor's Certification Board. Dr. Clayton lives with his wife, Cathy, and their three children in Piedmont, Oklahoma.

Photo Credits

Cover photo by Stuart Rabinowitz; p. 17 © Greg Smith/ Gamma-Liaison; p. 20 © Alice Q. Hargrave/Gamma-Liaison; pp. 23, 26 © Gamma-Liaison; p. 29 © Jean Marc Giboux/ Gamma-Liaison; all other photos by Stuart Rabinowitz.